The Frugal Way to Natural Beauty

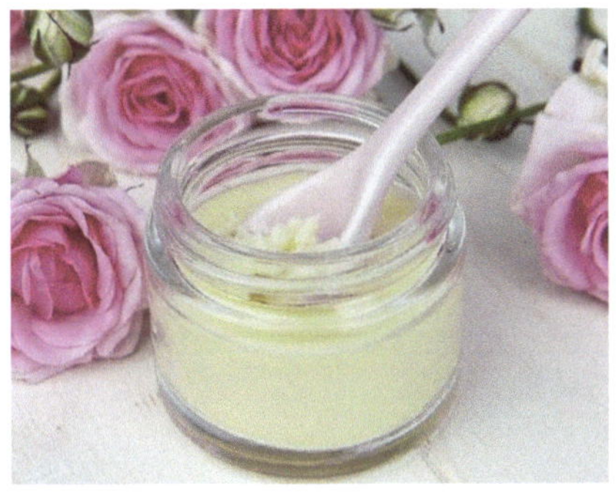

Michelle Tricomi

INTRODUCTION

Thank you for your purchase. I wish you the best of luck in your journey to natural beauty products!

If you have been searching in the stores or online you quickly come to the tough realization that natural or organic equals expensive, but it doesn't have to be! There are some very simple products that can be used in your beauty regimen that have the same benefits, if not more, to those high end products in the stores!

In this book I will give you some amazing ways to get that beautiful skin that you have been longing for without the harsh ingredients or price!

COCONUT OIL

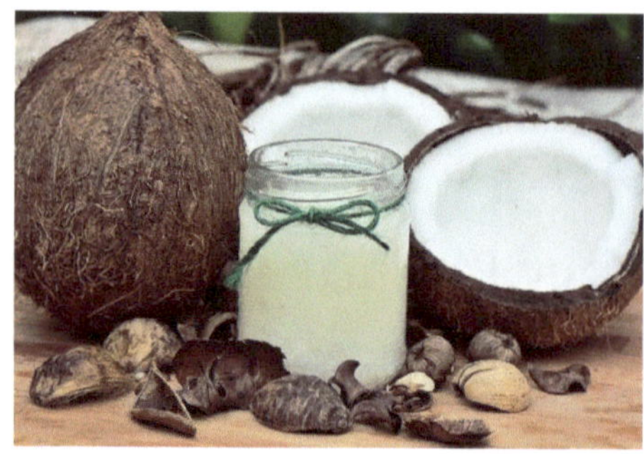

I'm jumping right in with this amazing ingredient because it is incredible and effective on its own as well as mixed with other ingredients to create an incredible beauty product that helps with wrinkles, dry skin, acne and many other common skin problems that people are prone to!

Coconut oil is a medium chain fatty acid. It has small molecules that allow it to penetrate the skin and is rich in fatty acids such as capric acid, caprylic acid and lauric acid. The lauric acid in coconut oil has **anti-fungal** and **anti-bacterial** properties. Coconut oil can be used to help heal infections, such as athlete's foot and ringworm, as well as aid in healing cuts and minor burns. The fatty acids have **disinfectant** and **anti-microbial** properties. Coconut oil is high in vitamin E, which is known for its skin healing properties. The triglycerides in coconut oil help to keep moisture from escaping which aids in retaining softness in the skin. Like coconuts themselves, coconut oil is rich in many proteins. These proteins keep skin healthy and rejuvenated, both internally and externally. Proteins also contribute to cellular health and tissue repair, along with a wide range of other essential activities within the body.

Here are some great ways to mix coconut oil with other other ingredients to help combat tough skin conditions or maintain your naturally beautiful skin.

1. When mixed with honey and lavender essential oil it can be used as a calming and moisturizing facial mask.
2. When mixed with sugar (for your face) or salt (for rougher parts) it makes an incredibly moisturizing and exfoliating scrub.
3. When mixed with baking soda it makes an incredible cleanser.
4. When used by itself it is an incredible

moisturizer for normal dry skin as well as a soother for a sunburn. A tiny amount massaged into your scalp will help with dandruff and frizzy hair.

5. When mixed with a few drops of your favorite essential oil it makes a great deodorant.
6. When mixed with baking soda and peppermint essential oil it turns into an incredible whitening toothpaste!

This list could go on and on, however, the point is that coconut oil is fairly inexpensive and can be used for so many amazing things when it comes to beauty!

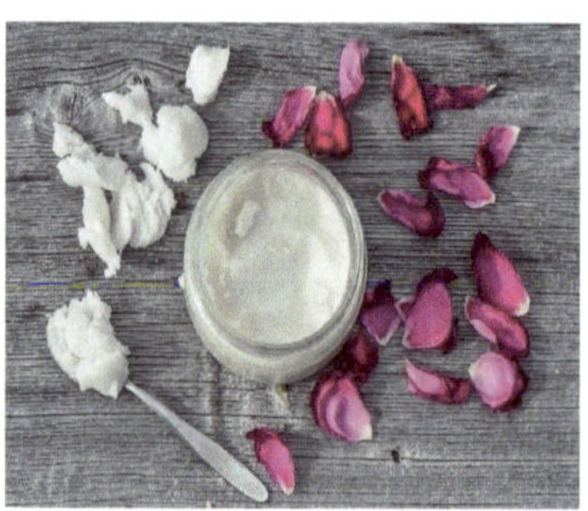

ESSENTIAL OILS 101

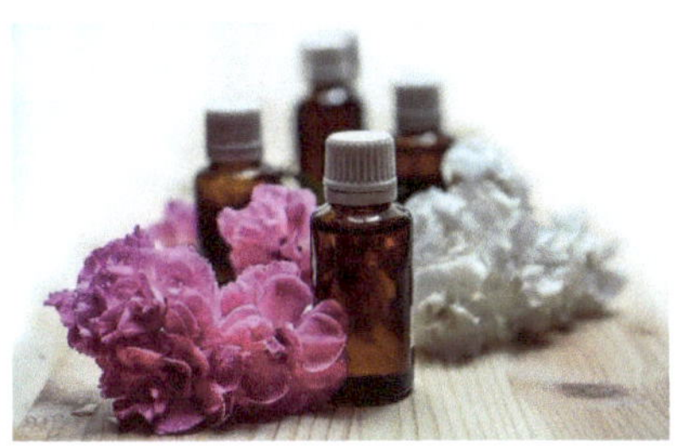

Essential oils are key when it comes to beauty at home! While not as inexpensive as coconut oil they still serve so many purpose in skincare and a little goes a long way. The initial investment is big but the joy keeps going and going for a long time!! When choosing what brand of essential oils to use please be aware that A LOT of companies claim to be all natural and pure when, in reality, they do not practice the appropriate cultivation methods that they should. You can do your own research on this but don't hesitate to ask questions to see how they cultivate their flowers and what other additives they may be using! As a rule, avoid buying essential oils from a company that prices all of its oils the same. The process of extraction can vary enormously from one plant to the next. Pricing like this suggests that the oils are either synthetic or of low quality. Ultimately, the price of an oil should be based on how much of the raw material is needed to produce it.

A few other things to look out for are:

- Avoid essential oils that have been diluted with vegetable oil. To test this, place a couple of drops on a piece of paper. If the drop leaves an oily ring, it likely contains vegetable oil.

- Choose oils from companies that list the Latin name and common name on the label as well as the country of origin.

- Essential oils should be sold in dark amber or blue glass bottles. Clear glass allows unfiltered light to enter and can cause the oil to spoil.

- Never buy essential oils in plastic bottles as the oils can dissolve plastic and contaminate the product.

Now that you know what to look for when purchasing your essential oils, lets have some fun on how they are beneficial as well as how to use them for skincare!

Lavender oil is the one oil that I suggest no one goes without! The smell alone is enough to have it on hand as well as the way it helps you relax and your body adapt to stress but it also has great benefits for your skin! It helps regenerate skin cells, which is amazing for mature skin, sun spots, and scarring. It is a great oil for all skin

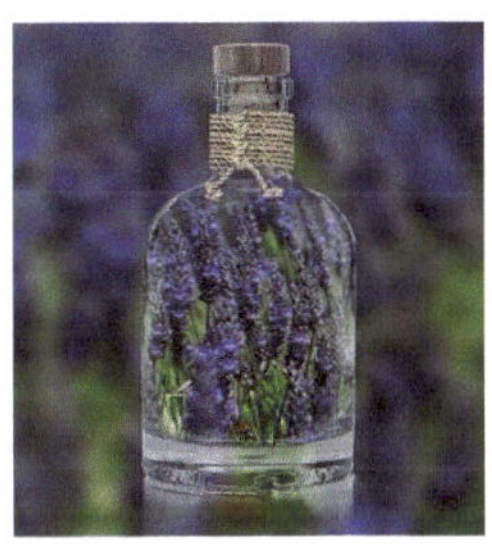 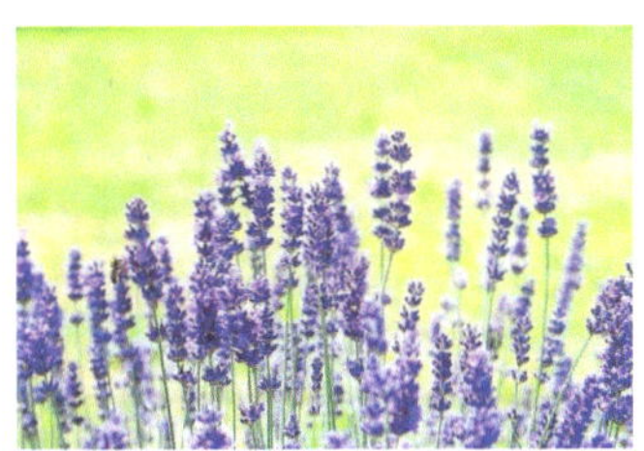

types!

Ways to use Lavender Essential Oil:

- Diffuse for mental clarity, peaceful sleep and relaxation.

- Apply directly to the temple to relieve headaches.

- Apply to acne.

- Add 1-2 drops to coconut oil for chapped skin and lips.

- Add directly to the skin for bug bite relief.

- Add a few drops to a carrier oil for sunburn relief.

Tea Tree Oil is one of the more well-known essential oils for acne-prone skin. It has antibacterial properties that help ward off acne-causing bacteria and assist in healing wounds. It also helps to regulate oil production, which can decrease the severity and incidence of breakouts.

Ways to use Tea Tree Essential Oil:

- Add to shampoo to lessen dandruff symptoms and to prevent LICE!

- Add to organic facial cream or toner to help fight acne.

- Add to toenails to combat fungus.

- Add to a carrier oil and apply to Athlete's feet.

- Add 1-2 drops to your laundry to kill bacteria on your clothes and in the washer. (Not skin care, I know, but too interesting to leave out!)

Patchouli Oil is particularly great for aging skin. It promotes new cell growth and smooths the appearance of fine lines and wrinkles. It also has antiseptic, anti fungal, and antibacterial properties so it can also benefit skin conditions such as eczema, dermatitis, psoriasis, and acne.

Ways to use Patchouli Essential Oil:

- Add 3-5 drops into a carrier oil for a therapeutic massage.

- Add 10 drops into your bath water.

- Add 4 drops to water or witch hazel for a natural bug spray.

- Add 5 drops to 1 TBSP of carrier oil or unscented organic moisturizer for facial cream.

- Add 4 drops to 2 oz of water in a spray bottle for a chemical free deodorant.

- Add 3-5 drops to a diffuser filled with water for a peaceful transition to sleep!

Ylang Ylang Essential Oil helps to control oil production and minimize breakouts. It also helps regenerate skin cells, smoothing fine lines and improving skin elasticity. Another great essential oil for every skin type.

Ways to use Ylang Ylang Essential Oil:

- Add 1-2 drops to lightly scented shampoo and conditioner to promote hair growth.

- Add 5 drops to chamomile tea for use as a calming facial toner.

- Add 3-4 drops to coconut oil in a roller-ball and rub on the abdomen to balance hormones.

- Massage a single drop into a sore muscle area to relieve tension.

- Add to a diffuser for stress relief.

Rose Essential Oil is especially great for dry or aging skin. Researchers have found that it contains several therapeutic compounds known to promote healing, especially antimicrobial and anti-inflammatory compounds. As a result, rose essential oil helps refine skin texture and tone, and can be helpful with managing skin conditions such as psoriasis and dermatitis. Very calming and also boasts an amazing scent!

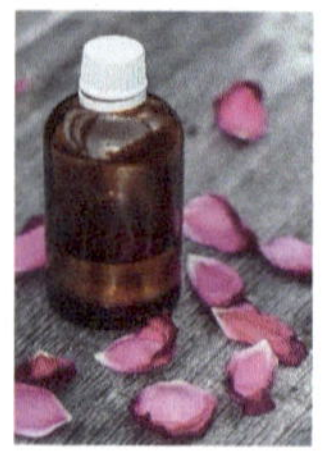 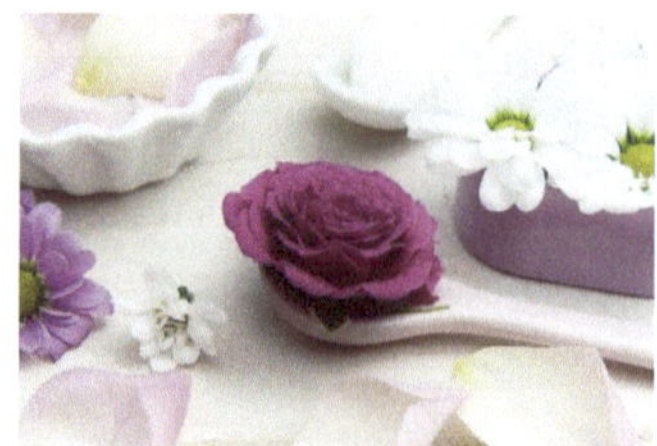

Ways to use Rose Essential Oil:

- Add 1-2 drops to the abdomen to relieve menstrual cramps.

- Add 1-2 drops to wounds and insect bites to prevent infections.

- Add 3-4 drops to water or witch hazel in a spray bottle for a calming and balancing facial toner.

- Add 1-2 drops to stretch marks and scars to reduce appearance.

Neroli Essential Oil is great for oily, sensitive, and mature skin. It helps to smooth fine lines and tone sagging skin. This rejuvenating oil contains a natural chemical called citral, which helps regenerate cells. It is said to be very good at preventing and healing stretch marks, as well. Its antiseptic properties also balance oil production and shrink the appearance of pores without drying skin.

Ways to use Neroli Essential Oil:

- Add to diffuser to lower blood pressure.

- Add a few drops to bath water to relieve PMS symptoms.

- Add 3-4 drops to lotion or oil to reduce stretch marks.

- Add 1-2 drops to a damp cotton ball and dab on areas to treat acne.

- Add 3 drops to facial cream to regenerate skin.

Myrrh Essential Oil has amazing anti aging benefits! It has strong anti-inflammatory properties that help improve skin tone, firmness, and skin elasticity, reducing the appearance of fine lines and wrinkles. Myrrh oil can also help heal sun damage, chapped skin, rashes, and eczema.

Ways to use Myrrh Essential Oil:

- Add a few drops to water and use as a mouth rinse to protect gums and freshen breath.

- Add 2-4 drops to a cool, wet towel to create a homemade compress for skin sores and wounds.

- Add 3-4 drops to a diffuser to help relieve stress and combat upper respiratory infections.

Geranium Essential Oil helps regulate oil production and reduces acne breakouts. It also helps improve skin elasticity and tighten skin, reducing the appearance of wrinkles. It promotes blood circulation to the areas where it is applied, helping to heal bruises, broken capillaries, burns, cuts, dermatitis, eczema, ringworm, and other skin conditions. This is an amazing essential oil to have on hand!

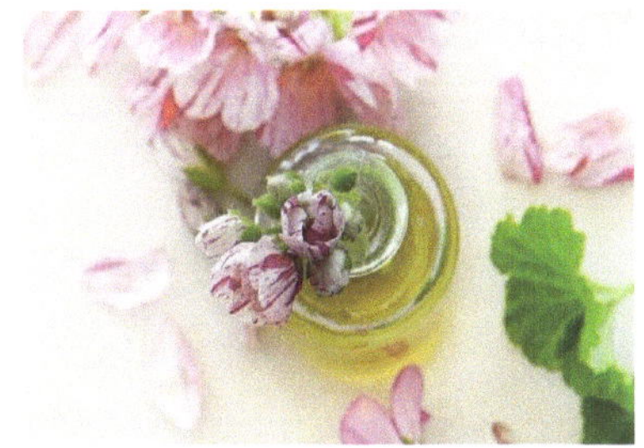 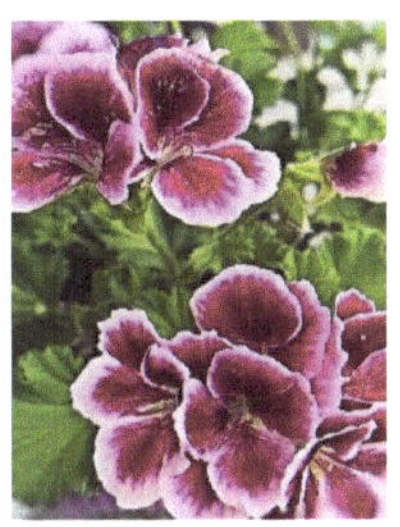

Ways to use Geranium Essential Oil:

- Add 2 drops to face lotion and use 2 times daily to help diminish wrinkles.

- Add 5 drops to a spray bottle with 5 tablespoons of water for a chemical free deodorant.

- Add 1-2 drops to cuts or wounds and cover with gauze to help with healing.

Frankincense Essential Oil has antibacterial and anti-inflammatory benefits, making it great for acne-prone skin. It is also a natural toner, decreasing the appearance of pores and evening skin-tone. It encourages new cell growth, helping to tighten skin and reduce wrinkles and the appearance of scars. It also helps soothe chapped, dry skin. It is perfect for all skin types!

Ways to use Frankincense Essential Oil:

- Add to itchy skin for instant relief.

- Apply 1-2 drops to brittle nails to help strengthen them.

- Add 1-2 drops to a carrier oil and apply to soles of feet to strengthen your immune system.

- Add 3-4 drops to a carrier oil and rub on abdomen to relieve gas and bloating.

- Apply directly to a wart for 1-2 weeks.

Carrot Seed Essential Oil has a rejuvenating effect on the skin. It not only works to help smooth skin, but assists with cell regeneration. It can aid in reducing scars and improve the tone of aging skin. It is also rich in antioxidants, helping to neutralize inflammation and wrinkle causing free radicals.

Ways to use Carrot Seed Essential Oil:

- Add 3-5 drops to 1 Tsp of a carrier oil and apply to skin in a circular motion to help prevent dryness and discoloration.

- Apply 10-12 drops directly to the scalp and massage for 5 minutes before going to bed to reduce dandruff. Wash out the next morning.

- Add 1-2 drops to your pillow to

promote restful sleep.

- Add to a diffuser for an amazing smell!

As an end note to this amazing chapter I need to let you know that ANY product that you make using essential oils NEEDS to be stored in a glass container as the oils will melt the plastic. The plastic will leach chemicals into your products, which wouldn't make any sense while you are trying to make products for exactly that reason.

BODY AND FACE SCRUB

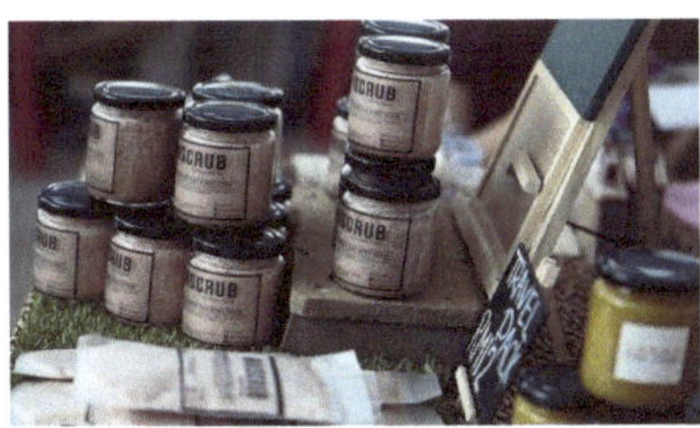

One of the easiest ways to save money when looking for beauty care products is to make your own scrub! There are so many variations from therapeutic to healing that are very easy and inexpensive to make at home. Above all the BEST benefit is that you can determine what goes in to your scrubs and can make the most all natural products at home!

Whether it is a body scrub or a facial scrub you will only want to use it 1-2 times a week to exfoliate and smooth your skin.

For rough skin, such as feet and elbows, you can use salt as the base as it is more abrasive. For more sensitive areas, such as your face and other skin, you should try white sugar or brown sugar as the base.

As I am writing this, it is winter in New England, so I'll start out with some combinations for colds and congestion. By using them in the shower when you are experiencing cold symptoms you are not only exfoliating but also relieving congestion!

The best way to make scrub is with coconut oil, salt or sugar and essential oils. The coconut oil really softens your skin, the salt or sugar exfoliate and the essential oils make it smell fantastic! So, naturally, a scrub made with eucalyptus, peppermint, spearmint or menthol mixed with the steam from your shower will not only exfoliate your skin but also clear your congestion and help you ease into the day!

Other scrubs that come to mind in the winter are:

Chocolate Mint – Salt, Coconut oil, cocoa powder and peppermint oil. This makes an amazing gift as well!

Vanilla Coffee – Salt, Coconut oil, coffee grinds (actually help with cellulite) and Vanilla.

Gingerbread Cookie – Sugar, Coconut oil, Ginger (oil or powder), Cinnamon (be careful if you have sensitive skin), Clove essential oil.

Vanilla Cookie – Sugar (brown or white), Coconut oil, vanilla extract

Now let's talk spring and summer!! So many fun ways to use those fresh fruits and herbs for more than just snacks!

Lemongrass & Ginger – Salt or Sugar, Coconut Oil, Lemongrass Essential Oil (stimulates circulation and keeps the bugs away!), Ginger Oil (great for stimulating digestion)!

Rosemary & Spearmint – Salt, Coconut oil, Rosemary Essential Oil (antiseptic and antimicrobial properties to help acne-prone skin), Spearmint Oil (pain relieving properties)!

Cucumber & Mint – Salt, Coconut Oil, Cucumber Puree (unpeeled as it adds extra antioxidants to the skin), Peppermint Essential Oil (it smells fantastic)!

Coconut & Lime – Salt or Sugar, Coconut Oil, Shredded Coconut, Lime juice or essential oil! This scrub SCREAMS summer and will put you in a fantastic mood!

Pineapple & Coconut – Sugar, Coconut Oil, shredded coconut, Pineapple Puree

Watermelon & Kiwi – Sugar, Coconut Oil, Watermelon puree or flavoring, Kiwi juice and seeds

The last few scrubs are reserved for my favorite scented time of year... FALL!

Pumpkin Spice – Sugar, Coconut Oil, Pumpkin Pie Spice, vanilla

Apple Spice – Brown Sugar, Coconut Oil, Apple Pie Spice, Vanilla

Maple Sugar – Brown and White Sugar, Coconut Oil, Maple Syrup

Oatmeal Cookie – Brown Sugar, Coconut Oil, Oats

(blended to a powder), vanilla

Cranberry – Salt, Coconut oil and whole cranberries! Puree the cranberries and add other ingredients!

I will end this chapter by adding that any of the recipes can be made with salt or sugar as well as any other oil, if you are not a fan of (or allergic to) coconut! Also be careful with cinnamon as sometimes it is harsh on skin. If that is the case, use an oil not the powder. I'm sure you will come up with your own recipes as the options are truly endless! Enjoy being creative and saving money in the process.

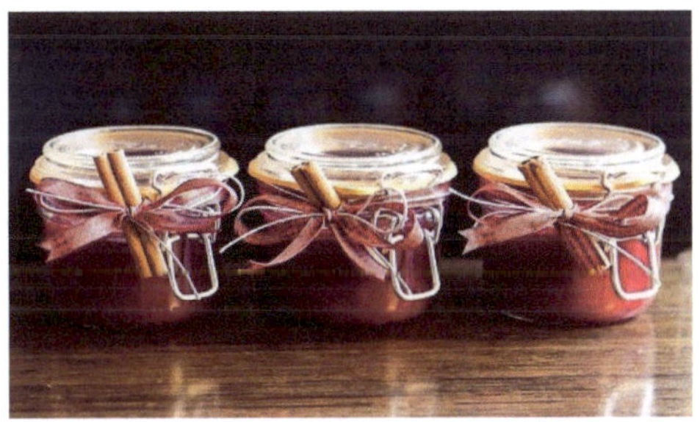

NATURAL FACIAL CARE

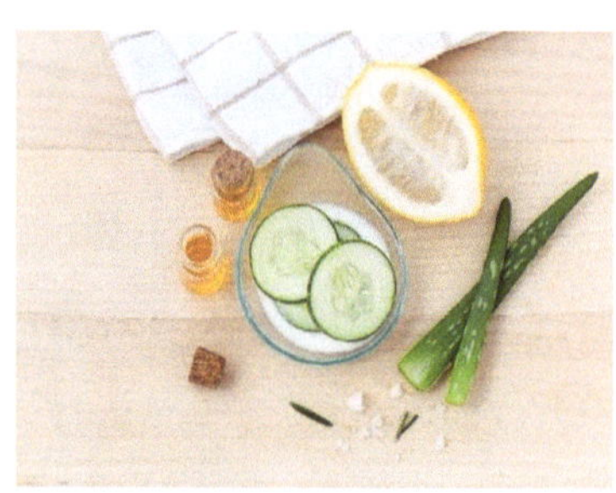

Let's dive right into Facial Care because it tends to be the most expensive beauty product out there, not to mention the amount of choices there are for it! Everyone knows, for the most part, what kind of skin they have, whether it be oily, combination, dry, acne-prone or naturally gorgeous! Regardless of what type of skin you have, finding the right products for your skin can be daunting.

The first, and most important, facial care practice is cleansing. How you cleanse your skin, how often and with what are very important steps in the natural beauty process. Cleansing can be as simple as Coconut oil and baking soda! Both bring forth cleansing properties as well as help fight acne! It won't be the best for everyone but for the cost, it is definitely worth a try!

Another variation of this is to add witch hazel and tea tree oil in place of the baking soda. Tea tree is also great at fighting acne but can be harsh on sensitive skin.

Another **homemade facial cleanser** recipe is: ½ cup liquid castile soap such as Dr. Bronners, ½ cup rose water and 10 drops of rose hip seed oil mixed with 1 tsp of a carrier oil(coconut, olive, almond or jojoba).

The next step to take after cleansing is to tone! Toners are extremely easy to make (and super expensive to purchase) using witch hazel, a few drops of essential oil like tea tree, rose hip oil or something more calming such as lavender. Additions to this are to add cucumber, lavender sprigs or rose petals. You will feel like you are at the spa, not to mention, it will serve as a gorgeous spa like bathroom decor!

Moisturizer is one of the most expensive things to purchase, especially when it is organic or all natural! It does take a little longer to make, however, it will save you A LOT of money!

The easiest one I have found thus far is made with my favorite ingredient as well as Vitamin E oil and Lavender Essential Oil! Coconut oil is great for anti-aging and is anti-fungal, anti-bacterial and anti-microbial! Vitamin E oil is known for reducing scar tissue and acne. It also helps to hold this moisturizer together as well as serve as a preservative! Lavender Essential Oil is a well known antioxidant, helping to rid skin of free radicals.

Here is the moisturizer recipe:
½ Cup Coconut Oil
1 teaspoon liquid Vitamin E oil
12 drops of Lavender Essential Oil

Melt the coconut by placing in a bowl of warm water. Add in the Vitamin E and Lavender Oil. Mix it all and let it set. Whip with a fork if desired. When the coconut oil solidifies you will have your first homemade moisturizer! I always suggest storing beauty products, especially when made with essential oil, in glass jars. Mason jars are perfect as well as super cute!

Another fairly simple one to make uses aloe vera which is amazing for skin, beeswax as a stabilizer, almond oil, coconut oil and Essential Oil!

Here is another moisturizer recipe:
1 cup Aloe Vera Gel (be careful with added ingredients and make sure it is a gel!)
¾ ounce beeswax (many ways to purchase but make sure it is not for candle making or scented)
¼ cup Almond Oil
¼ cup Coconut Oil
10 drops of Essential Oil (lavender, grapefruit, tea tree etc.... be sure to test on your skin first)

Start by melting the beeswax, coconut oil and almond oil (use a chocolate melting pot or double broiler). Let cool (at least an hour) and put in blender. Mix the essential oil into the cup of aloe vera gel. Start the blender again and slowly pour in the mixture as it whips. That's it! Another great moisturizer that you can add your own ingredients and touches to! Jojoba or olive oil can replace the other oils if there are allergies, although it will not be as thick.

One final recipe that I can share that does not use my favorite ingredient uses Almond Oil, Aloe Vera Gel, Apricot Kernel Oil, Beeswax or Jojoba wax and essential oil such as lemon and orange!

Final Moisturizer recipe:
2 tbsp Sweet Almond Oil
1/3 cup Aloe Vera Gel
2 tbsp Apricot Kernel Oil
1 tbsp Jojoba or Beeswax
10 drops of essential oil

Combine Almond and Apricot oils as well as wax in a glass bowl and place in a half-filled pan of water. Leave on low until the wax melts. Let cool. Add essential oils to the aloe vera gel. Slowly pour the gel into the oil/wax mixture using a hand mixer. Continue whipping until it gets to a buttery consistency.

Just because I'm having fun I will also throw in some recipes for face masks! **Why not right?** These are extremely easy to make and you will definitely feel like you are at the spa. Pampering yourself from the comfort of your own home is truly and perfectly satisfying!

The following 3 combinations use Turmeric powder and are simply amazing!

For **acne-prone** skin mix 1 tsp turmeric, 1 spoonful Manuka honey and 1 tsp cinnamon. Leave on for

10 minutes

For **brightening** qualities mix 1 spoonful of yogurt, 1 tsp turmeric and a few drops of lemon. Leave on for 20 minutes.

For **smoothing** Fine Lines and Wrinkles mix 1 tsp turmeric and 1 spoonful of coconut oil (couldn't resist)! Leave on for 20 minutes.
A few fun facial masks using banana:

For **Acne-prone** mix 2 tbsp mashed banana, 1 tbsp baking soda and ½ tbsp fresh lemon juice. Leave on for 10-12 minutes. Use twice a week.

For **smoothing** wrinkles mix 2 tbsp mashed banana, 1 tbsp yogurt and ½ tbsp fresh lemon juice. Leave on for 20-25 minutes. Use 3-4 times a week.

For **brightening** Skin mix 2 tbsp mashed banana and 1 tbsp honey. Leave on for 20-30 minutes. Use twice a week.

There are so many variations to these recipes. You need to experiment and educate yourself on what works best for skincare and specifically what works best for your skin! In the next chapter you will learn a little more about why making your own products are so much better and what ingredients to stay away from if you do purchase pre-made products.

NATURAL MAKEUP

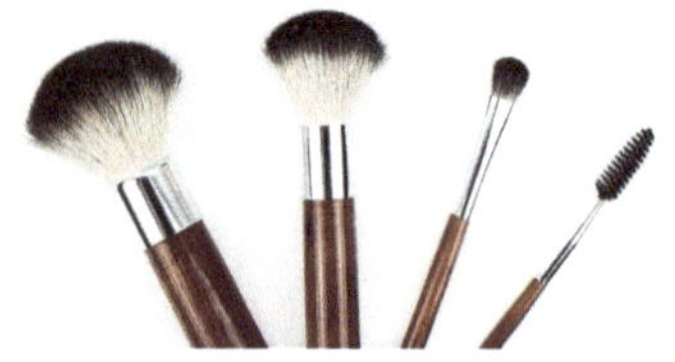

Makeup is something that I have struggled with for years! The bigger companies are much more inexpensive but add an unsettling amount of chemicals. The organic makeup is more expensive but is so much better for your skin, however, may still contain ingredients that are not the greatest for your skin! Let's use this time to give you a list of ingredients to avoid and then I'll give you a few recipes to try at home!

Here are the top ingredients to avoid:

Phthalates are found in many products and have been known to damage liver and kidneys, cause birth defects, decrease sperm count and play a role in early breast development in both girls and boys! They are used as plasticizers to increase flexibility and durability in plastic and can be found in adhesives for vinyl floors!

Parabans (ALL OF THEM) The FDA acknowledges several studies linking parabens, which mimic estrogen, to breast cancer, skin cancer and decreased sperm count, but has not ruled that it is harmful. According to the European Commission's Scientific Committee on Consumer Products, longer chain parabens like propyl and butyl paraben and their branched counterparts, isopropyl and isobutylparabens, may disrupt the endocrine system and cause reproductive and developmental disorders. Look for ingredients with the suffix "-paraben" as well paraben-free products will be labeled as such. (www.EWG.org)

Talc is a powdered native, hydrous magnesium silicate, sometimes containing a small portion of aluminum silicate. Talc can be contaminated with asbestos fibers, posing risks for respiratory toxicity and cancer. Studies by the National Toxicology Panel demonstrated that cosmetic-grade talc free of asbestos is a form of magnesium silicate that also can be toxic and carcinogenic. (www.EWG.org)

Formaldehyde is used in paint, adhesives, disinfectants and TOBACCO! It has been known to cause respiratory issues, burn the skin, cause skin irritations and cause cancer. Most commonly found in nail polish!

Synthetic fragrance The word "fragrance" or "parfum" on the product label represents an undisclosed mixture of various scent chemicals and ingredients used as fragrance dispersants such as diethyl phthalate.

Fragrance mixes have been associated with allergies, dermatitis, respiratory distress and potential effects on the reproductive system. (www.EWG.org)

Dioxins According to the U.S. Environmental Protection Agency (EPA), dioxins a family of toxic chemicals that share a similar chemical structure and induce harm through a similar mechanism. Dioxins have been characterized by EPA as likely human carcinogens and are anticipated to increase the risk of cancer at background levels of exposure. (www.EWG.org)

Sulfates are used in car washes, garage floor cleaners, engine de-greasers and 90% of skin care products! They can lead to eye damage, depression, skin irritation and many other problems!

Toluene A volatile petrochemical solvent and paint thinner, toluene is a potent neurotoxicant that acts as an irritant, impairs breathing, and causes nausea. Mother's exposure to toluene vapors during pregnancy may cause developmental damage in the fetus. In human epidemiological studies and in animal studies toluene has been also associated with toxicity to the immune system and a possible link to blood cancer such as malignant lymphoma. Can also be called Benzene! (www.EWG.org)

Now that we know what to avoid when purchasing makeup let's take a look at the possibility of making it at home so we know it is safe!

It all starts with a strong foundation so why not make a **face powder** you can trust....right?
Light Powder: 2tbsp arrowroot powder, ½ tsp cocoa powder, ¼ tsp cinnamon

Medium Powder: 2 tbsp arrowroot powder, 1 ½ tsp cocoa powder, ¼ tsp cinnamon

Dark Powder: 2 tbsp arrowroot powder, 1 tbsp cocoa powder, ¼ tsp cinnamon

AMAZING RIGHT!? Who would have ever guessed it could be that easy, inexpensive and good for you to make your own! I will add that cinnamon may not work for everyone so definitely test it on your skin first. Also make sure your face is well moisturized before applying and spritz on some toner to set it! It does make a bit of a mess on your shirt but brushes off easily!

While you already have the arrowroot powder from making your foundation powder try it in your **blush** and **eye shadow** recipes as well! Use powders such as beet root, hibiscus and peach powders to make the right shade for you. For darker shades add some cocoa powder in as well!

How about some super easy **eye shadow**?
Shades of brown: mix different amounts of arrowroot powder and cocoa powder.
Shades of green: use green clay or spirulina, again adding in arrowroot powder for the lighter shades.
Shades of Gray: use activated charcoal and arrowroot powder.
Shades of Orange: use Saffron and beetroot juice as well as turmeric (Turmeric can stain skin so be careful with it)
Shades of Purple: Rose Clay and Alkanet.

Eye liner and mascara you say.... DONE!

Mascara: 2 tsp aloe vera gel, 10 capsules of activated charcoal, 1/8 tsp Vitamin E oil, a pinch of bentonite clay and an empty mascara bottle that can be bought on Amazon!

Eye Liner: 1/5 tsp glycerin, 3 caplets of activated charcoal. Mix together and go! Its more of a gel than a pencil!

I simply cannot forget lip color! While I don't wear a colored lipstick myself I am adding in a lip gloss recipe as well!

Lipstick: Beeswax pastilles, 1 tsp shea butter or cocoa butter (yum) and 1 tsp coconut oil as the base and then add in your color. Melt beeswax, coconut oil and butter in a glass jar in a small pot of boiling water. When melted add the color choices you would like!

Red hues: 1/8 tsp of beet root powder or 1 drop of natural red food coloring

Brown/Tan Hues: ¼ teaspoon cocoa powder, tiny pinch of cinnamon or turmeric

Feel free to add a few drops of essential oil in as well, because, well... WHY NOT!

Lip Gloss: Coconut oil (surprise, surprise) and your favorite essential oil or flavor in powder form such as cocoa or coffee! Melt coconut oil, add flavor or color (using above blush and eye shadow ideas) and let sit to solidify. There are a ton of options on amazon for containers and its so easy to make you could give as gifts as well!

That is it! A whole lesson in makeup and why it is more beneficial to make your own. Most likely everything can be purchased online but you could also find most everything at an all natural market around you. If you choose to purchase pre-made products please take some time, read labels and educate yourself about the ingredients. A great website to help understand more about harmful ingredients is EWG.org! They give you the best products with the least chemicals and even have their own line, which I haven't tried but I'm sure is amazing.

Michelle Tricomi

HAIR CARE

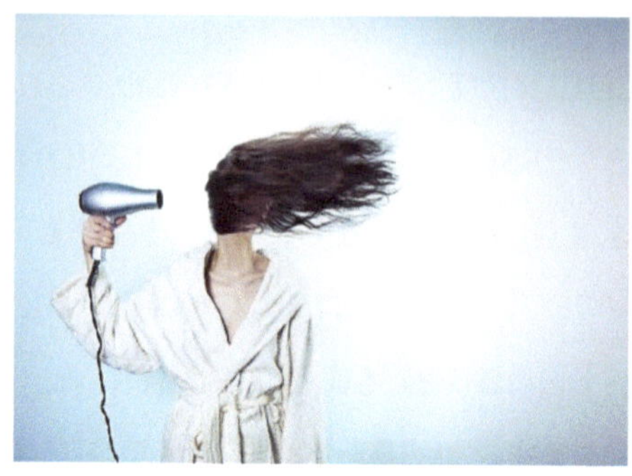

Shampoo, Conditioner, Hair Gel and Scalp Treatments... OH MY!

Do you ever wish your hair could smell and look amazing without adding chemicals to it? Wouldn't it be amazing to focus on a little mindfulness while taking a shower because your are in love with the way your shower products smell? NOW YOU CAN! By making your own products you are not only saving yourself money and a life full of toxic chemicals but you are also able to make exactly what you want and don't have to settle with a certain smell or feel that you are not crazy about?

Here is your chance! Take a peek at these super simple recipes for shampoo, conditioner, scalp treatments, gel and hairspray...there is sure to be a few that you are going to love and make all the time!

Let's start out with a fancier recipe just for fun!

Rosemary Mint Shampoo:

6 oz Aloe Vera Gel

3 Tbsp Olive Oil

10 Tbsp Baking Soda

20 Drops Rosemary Oil

10 Drops Peppermint Oil

Glass Jar

Mix all ingredients in a glass container and shake well before each use. Use the same amount your normally would and massage into your scalp and rinse well. DONE!

Rosemary Mint Conditioner:

¼ cup Coconut Oil

2 Tbsp Shea Butter

2 tsp Argan Oil

10 drops Rosemary Oil

6 drops Peppermint Oil

Melt Coconut oil and shea butter until it is liquid, allow to cool then add in essential oils and argan oil. Store in airtight glass container.   Before shampoo slowly work it up to your roots and let sit for 5 minutes. Shampoo to remove excess oils resulting in super soft shiny hair. Obviously not meant for already oily hair and scalp.

Moisturizing Shampoo:
1 cup Dr. Bronner's Liquid Castile Soap
½ cup canned coconut milk
1 tbsp aloe vera gel
1 tsp carrier oil (avocado, jojoba, almond etc)
1 tsp magnesium gel
25 drops of your favorite essential oils
10 drops vitamin E
10 drops Argan Oil
5 drops Carrot Seed Oil

Blend well using an immersion blender or by shaking vigorously in a glass jar. Store in a 16 ounce glass pump bottle for easy use. Peppermint and rosemary are amazing to stimulate hair growth.

Moisturizing Conditioner:

1 cup distilled water
2 tsp guar gum
1 tbsp aloe vera gel
1 tsp carrier oil
1 tsp magnesium gel
10 drops Argan oil
10 drops Vitamin E oil
5 drops Carrot Seed Oil

In a glass jar mix the carrier oil, guar gum and essential oils. Then add distilled water and shake well. Store in a glass pump bottle for easy use.

Leave-In Conditioner:
¼ cup distilled water (or boiled tap water that has cooled
1 tbsp canned coconut milk
10 drops of essential oil (something that you don't mind smelling like all day!)

Whisk coconut milk, water and essential oils and pour into a glass spray bottle. Shake well before each use and spritz through damp hair, comb and style as usual! This should be stored in the refrigerator as it doesn't have preservatives. The best way to make is in small batches and use within a week. To save coconut milk for future use use an ice cube tray to freeze in 1 tbsp increments!

Let's talk about your scalp because, lets face it, A LOT of people suffer from dry scalp from time to time and the "treatments" for it are pretty harsh medicated shampoos. I talked earlier about dropping a few drops of tea tree oil into your shampoo for prevention as well as applying coconut oil over night but here is a nice mask that can help as well.

Scalp Detox:
1 tsp baking soda
1 tbsp olive oil
¼ tsp cinnamon
Mix together and massage into scalp in gentle circular motions. Wrap a shower cap around your scalp and hair. Leave on for 10-15 minutes. Shampoo and condition as usual.
*Massaging scalp will help stimulate your scalp, increase circulation and helps remove dead skin cells.

I cannot talk about your hair without giving you

recipes for hair spray and gel, so, here it goes!

Hair Gel:

3 tbsp aloe vera gel

½ – 1 tsp gelatin (start low and work your way up depending on the hold you are looking for)

1-2 drops of your favorite essential oil

Mix together in a glass jar and it will be fully ready within 24 hours. It can be used prior to then, however, may not be quite as much of a hold as you are looking for.

Hair Spray:

(Flexible Hold)

½ cup almost boiling water

1 tsp sugar

Mix together and pour into a glass spray bottle. Spray on hair and style usual

(Max Hold)

½ cup almost boiling water

2 tsp sugar

1 tsp salt

Mix together and pour into a glass spray bottle and style as usual.

I know what you are thinking..... gross my hair will be so sticky! Not true at all. It dries fast and adds great texture. Try it for yourself, you will be happy you did.

As this chapter comes to an end please know that there are so many variations of these recipes and a little tweaking to make it work the best for you. The main goal is to get the chemicals out and use natural products so that your hair can begin to detox and be the healthiest it can be. Adding different mixes of essential oils is a fun twist as well so that you never have the same exact recipe twice!

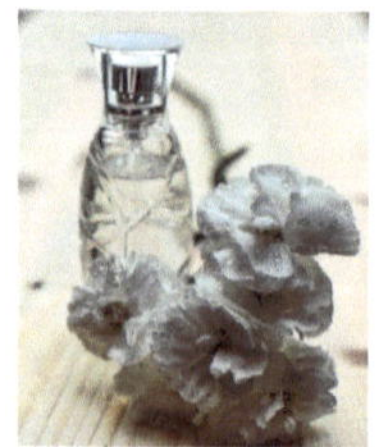 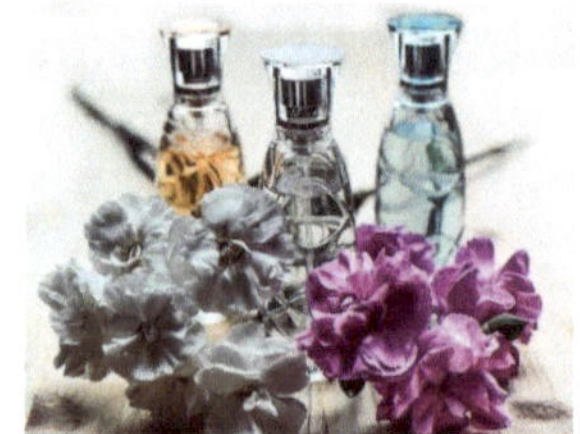

In closing, I hope that you can take some of these recipes and suggestions and start living the all natural lifestyle that you have been dreaming of. Natural doesn't always mean expensive so remember that EVERYTIME you are shopping for beauty products. It takes a little time and practice, however, the end result is a happy, healthy YOU as well as better products for your family.

If you are not up for the challenge of making your own products please make sure you are reading labels and researching ingredients. You will be surprised at the terrible things the bigger (and even smaller) companies are expecting you to put on your skin.

I hope you feel satisfied with the education and recipes found in this book and that you can create multiple Happy Spa Days at home for a fraction of the cost!

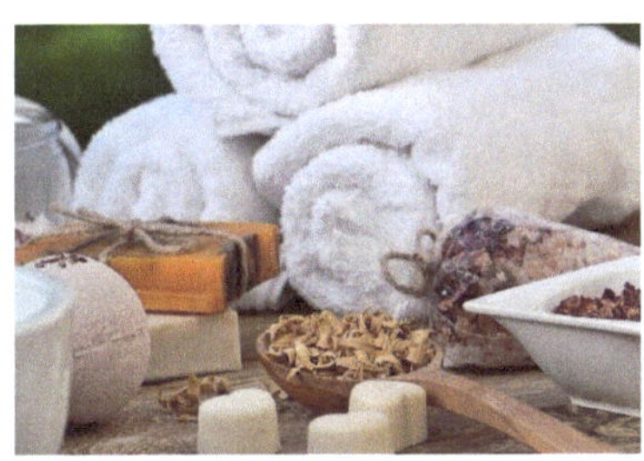

About the Author

I am a Wife, Mom, Sister, Daughter, Friend and lover of all things natural! I strive to learn more everyday about the ways I can provide my family with natural products and holistic practices. Some work for us and some don't. Some people get sick of hearing me try to educate them about what they should try instead of the over the counter medicine that they continue using with no changes. I've been called a hippie, a tree hugger and all out crazy with all of the natural ways I have chosen to live. I will never give it up, but also never push it on anyone. Your life is your choice but if I care about you I'm going to give it an honest effort to change a few things to healthy living. This book is something that is extremely important to me because we often times struggle with the high cost to be able to live an organic and natural life! I wanted to give people the foundation to switch to this lifestyle if they also believe it is an important change for them to make! I'm passionate about educating others and hope you enjoy this book and the books to come!

The Frugal Way to Natural Beauty